# *The Concise Guide to Baby-Sitting*

# THE
# FRANKLIN WATTS
# CONCISE GUIDE TO
# *Baby-Sitting*

by Rubie Saunders

*illustrated by Tomie de Paolo*

FRANKLIN WATTS, INC. • NEW YORK
1972

Library of Congress Cataloging in Publication Data

Saunders, Rubie.
    The Franklin Watts concise guide to baby-sitting.

    (The Franklin Watts concise guide series)
    SUMMARY: Suggests ways to enter the baby-sitting
business, methods for handling children of different
ages, safety precautions, and the possibilities of a
summer play school.
    Half title: The concise guide to baby-sitting.
    1. Baby sitters—Juvenile literature.  2. Children
—Care and hygiene—Juvenile literature.  [1. Baby
sitters]  I. De Paola, Thomas Anthony, illus.
II. Title.  III. Title: The concise guide to baby-
sitting.

HQ769.S27        649'.1'0248        71-188479
ISBN 0-531-02563-2

*To Mother, My Favorite Baby-sitter*

# Contents

# The Concise Guide to Baby-Sitting

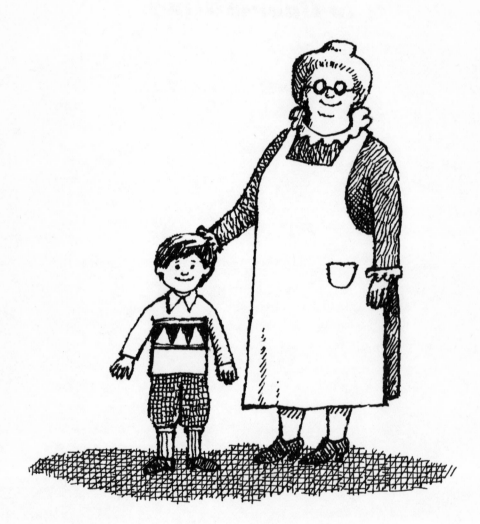

*Until fairly recently, baby-sitting fell to grandmothers and unmarried aunts who lived with the parents they sat for.*

# An Introduction to Baby-Sitting

Baby-sitting has been called the youngest profession, but it certainly isn't the newest. The task of temporarily taking care of someone else's children has been a very necessary one in every country, in every type of society, in every period of time. Until fairly recently, however, this task usually fell to grandmothers and unmarried aunts who lived with the parents they sat for.

But today's grandmothers are often very busy leading lives of their own, or else they live too far away to make sitting for their grandchildren practical. And modern unmarried women of all ages are now leading such full lives, both professionally and socially, that they simply do not have the time to entertain their nieces and nephews, except on special occasions.

When you add the fact that sleep-in servants today are extremely rare, it's easy to understand why teen-agers are in such great demand as baby-sitters. In bygone days, adults had all the baby-sitting jobs, but now the profession is open to young people who are eager to seize the opportunity to perform them. And who can blame them? The job of baby-sitting offers a great many advantages to those who are willing to give it a try.

# Why Baby-Sit?

While most youngsters baby-sit for the money they can earn, many soon discover that there are valuable fringe benefits to the job. They get to know a great deal about children: how they think; how they react in various situations; what can and cannot be expected of them at different ages. This is valuable information for baby-sitters to have when someday they have children of their own.

Since sitters are earning money, they soon learn how to handle it. And that's one lesson that can't be learned too soon! One experienced sitter, after spending her first earnings on records and accessories and other fad items, soon realized that it might be a better idea to save at least part of her money. By the time she was graduated from high school, she had enough saved in the bank to pay for her first year's tuition at college. And she is typical of thousands of baby-sitters who have used their income to give them a head start in the adult world.

By working in the homes of so many different people, sitters often get good ideas about what they personally like and dislike in styles of furniture, color combinations, and other aspects of interior decorating. They find out which electrical appliances work efficiently and which do not. They learn about good and bad housekeeping methods and many other household hints that can be helpful to them later on. Moreover, they can learn all this without snooping! All that's necessary is to use one's eyes and ears.

But perhaps the most immediate benefit, next to having money to spend, is learning how to apply for a job and how to sell one's talents to a prospective employer. The girl who is too shy to ring a neighbor's bell or pick up a telephone and say that she's available for baby-sitting, explaining what training and

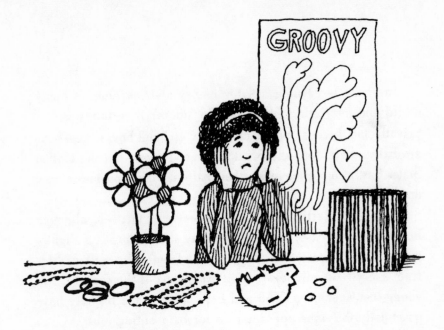

*One sitter, after spending her first earnings on records, accessories, and fad items, soon realized it might be better to save some of her money.*

experience she may have had, is not going to get any sitting jobs. And she'll have trouble later on — when she's ready for that full-time job after graduating from school — if she doesn't get to work now to overcome her shyness.

In addition to these advantages, baby-sitting can be a lot of fun. One sitter, who is an only child, enjoys her work because it makes her feel less lonely. Another, who wants to be a kindergarten teacher, finds working with toddlers a pure delight. Even youngsters who became sitters just for the money discovered that they enjoyed being around small children. One such sitter even went so far as to confess, "I think I'd sit even if I didn't get paid for it!"

If you think you'd like an adult career that brings you in close contact with children — teaching, certain types of social work, and medical careers, for example — baby-sitting is an excellent way to find out if you really have the patience and stamina required for this kind of work.

Just who is earning all this money and learning so many useful and interesting things as baby-sitters? It certainly isn't a private club, because practically every girl and boy — yes, boys are baby-sitters, too, and often very good ones — in the United States has, at one time or another, baby-sat for someone at least once.

The usual starting age is about twelve or thirteen, although in a few special cases a girl or boy may start sitting at a slightly younger age. These young people come from every walk of life; from every economic level; from every part of the country. The young teen-ager on a farm and her cousin in the big city have practically the same opportunities for baby-sitting jobs.

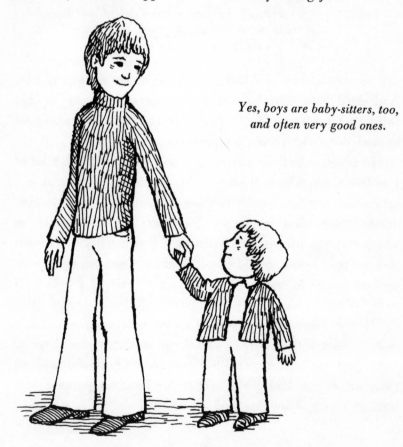

*Yes, boys are baby-sitters, too, and often very good ones.*

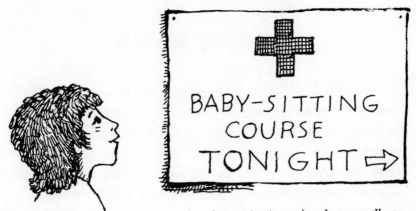

*Local organizations often have excellent courses on baby-sitting.*

## First Things First

The very first thing to do when you decide you'd like to be a baby-sitter is to take a course in child care if at all possible. Books and pamphlets on the subject are extremely helpful, but being in a class where you can have your questions answered on the spot will give you the confidence you'll need. After all, taking care of a child is a big responsibility, and knowing what you are doing will make the job easier for you.

Local chapters of the Red Cross, Y's, Scout Councils, and other organizations frequently have excellent courses aimed at prospective baby-sitters. Sometimes department stores offer such courses, too, and the home-economics department of many junior and senior high schools has them as well.

It makes it much easier to sell yourself to a would-be employer if you can show her a certificate proving you've taken and completed a baby-sitting course given by a responsible organization. Sometimes these courses are free; sometimes you have to pay for them. In either case, it's a good investment in both time and money.

7

# Finding a Job

The next question is, "Where do I find baby-sitting jobs?" The answer to that depends, to some extent, upon where you live. In small communities, it's easier for a thirteen-year-old to approach a neighbor or family friend and offer her services as a sitter. In larger towns, it may be necessary for the would-be sitter to advertise. This can be done in several different ways.

Classified ads in local newspapers aren't expensive, and they are a good way to let people know you are available. The ad should contain your address or phone number, or you can use a box number that the newspaper will provide.

It would be a good idea to limit the area in the town that you'll work in, especially if yours is a large city. Simply include in your ad the information that you're only interested in jobs in the north end of town or whatever area you happen to live in. This will automatically eliminate your having to spend a lot of time traveling to and from your jobs. This is very important, especially for nighttime sitting.

Supermarkets, churches, temples, and other places where large numbers of people congregate often have bulletin boards. A neatly written or typed notice on one or more of these can lead to baby-sitting jobs. Or similar notices can be put in the mailboxes of large apartment houses in your area or in the mailboxes of private homes.

Junior and senior high schools frequently have placement centers for all kinds of after-school jobs, and many young people make good use of this free service to find baby-sitting positions. Organizations that work with young people — Boy and Girl Scouts, 4H, Camp Fire Girls, Boys' and Girls' Clubs, Y's — sometimes have a central office where youngsters can register for jobs. Adults seeking part-time or temporary help — such as

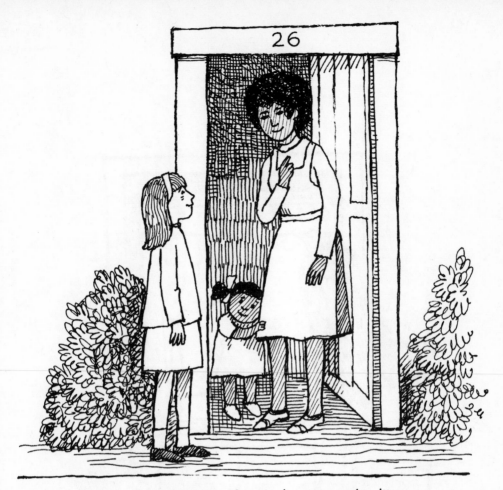

*In smaller communities, it's easier for a prospective sitter
to offer her services to a neighbor in person.*

mothers of small children — know they can find reliable assistants at such places.

Word-of-mouth advertising is another excellent way of letting people know you are available. Don't waste too much time telling your friends; instead, tell your neighbors and relatives, especially those with little children, that you are ready to sit for them. Learning how to sell yourself in this way is a valuable asset to have, and talking to people you already know and who know you is an easy way to start. If you sit back and wait for people to come to you with job offers, you're apt to have a long wait and an empty bank account.

**9**

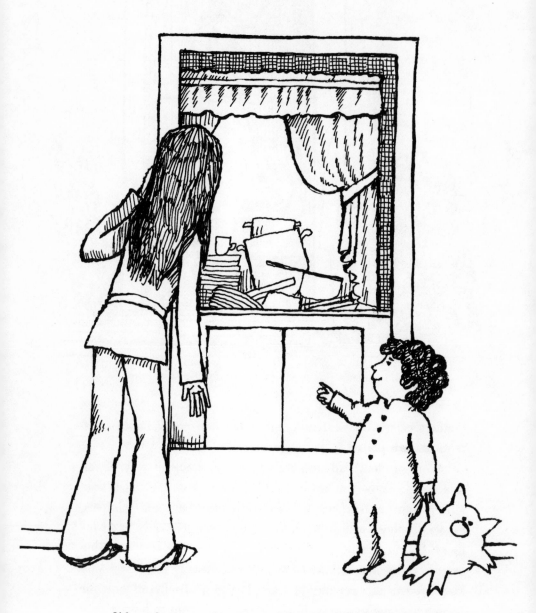

*If housekeeping tasks are included, a sitter can charge more.*

# How to Establish Rates

The next question facing beginners in this field is how much to charge. The best way to figure this out is to ask some experienced sitters what the going rate is in your community. Prices for baby-sitters differ a great deal from one part of the country to the next, but, generally speaking, about seventy-five cents an hour for daytime sitting and one dollar an hour for nighttime (after 6:00 P.M.) sitting is common. In some areas, nighttime sitting rates are lower than daytime rates. However, this is for straight baby-sitting; if some housekeeping tasks are included — such as washing the family's dinner dishes — the rates would be higher.

Sometimes the nighttime rate doesn't start until 10:00 P.M., but remember it's perfectly all right to charge more for night work than for working during the day.

There is such a wide difference in rates that in some parts of the country you may even find that daytime rates are higher than nighttime rates. This may be because there are more sitters available for evening jobs, and the competition has sent the prices down. That's why it is a good idea, before establishing your own rates, to find out from other sitters what the hourly rates are for both night and day. And make sure the prices you charge are in line with the other sitters' rates. If they are too high, no one will hire you; if they are too low, you'll be cheating yourself and making other sitters angry at you.

You may also discover, if you get your jobs through schools or some other agency, that the rates have been set for you. Don't let that be a cause for worry; they will probably be the same as the price independent sitters get. If there is a private baby-sitting agency in your community, you may have to pay them for the service of finding you a job. But since it probably won't be too hard for you to find a job on your own, you can save the expense of a private agency.

# Getting To and From Your Jobs

Getting to and from your jobs is an important part of the work. You should know in advance if your employer will pick you up and take you home. Usually, the sitter gets to the job on her own; that is, by some form of public transportation, or by occasionally having one of her parents drive her, or even by walking.

But getting home, especially after a nighttime job, can be a problem if you haven't made arrangements ahead of time. In most cases, senior high school and college boys and girls are often expected to find their own means of getting home, but younger girls are usually driven home by one of the parents of the child they are sitting for. However, if the sitter has to get home on her own, she is usually given extra money for carfare.

# Know Your Duties and Responsibilities

However you get that first baby-sitting job, it's always a good idea — and it makes a good impression on new customers — to meet with the mother and child (or children) before you actually go to work. It will only take about a half hour of your time, and it's time wisely spent.

At this session (which you don't charge for, incidentally) you ask the parents exactly what your duties will be. Do you have to prepare a meal for the child? If so, make sure you know how to do it. Find out exactly what the child may have to eat and where to find it. Check the stove so you'll know how to light the oven if necessary. Where are the pots and dishes you'll need?

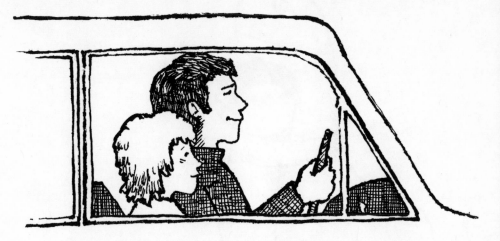

*Younger sitters are usually driven home
by one of the parents of the child they are sitting for.*

Does the child have a favorite dish that he eats from? This may seem like a lot of bother to go through to fix a snack for the six-year-old, but it will make your job much easier.

Some parents, when they're going out for the evening, leave the dinner dishes in the sink for the baby-sitter to wash. If this happens, you are perfectly justified to charge extra for that kind of service. Of course, if you are not specifically asked to wash them, you certainly don't have to do the dishes. But some sitters like to give a little extra service; it's entirely up to you.

For evening sitting, find out exactly what time the child has to go to bed. The closer you stick to his regular schedule the easier your job will be. Find out, too, if he is allowed to have liquids after dinner; whether he likes plain milk or chocolate milk; if there's a favorite toy he sleeps with.

The mother employing you will be favorably impressed if you take notes on all these details. Writing down this information will also save you from the embarrassment of confusing two entirely different children.

This preliminary interview is also the time to find out when the parents will return home and to make arrangements for your trip to and from their home.

13

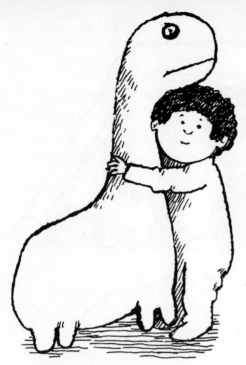

*Find out if there's a favorite toy your charge likes to sleep with.*

It is vitally important for you to know where the parents can be reached in an emergency or which neighbor to call if something comes up that you can't handle by yourself. And don't forget to ask for the phone number of the family doctor or the child's pediatrician.

For daytime sitting, you'll need to know if the youngster can be taken outdoors. If so, what extra clothing does he need? Where is it? If there's a playground or park nearby that you plan to take him to, ask if that's all right with his mother. Find out if the little one likes swings — some young children's stomachs get upset from the motion of a swing.

If you do plan to take the child outside, tell the mother exactly where and how long you intend to be. Will it be all right to buy some ice cream or cookies? In short, don't assume that it's okay to do something with someone else's child that you may be used to doing with your own kid brother or sister. The more specific questions you ask during the interview, the fewer chances you'll have to make mistakes when you're actually sitting with the child.

**14**

Try to get to know the child, too, during the interview. A good way to break the ice with a child of about two to four years old is to smile, say hello, and tell him your name. Then ask *his* name, but don't pounce on him. Remember you're much bigger than he is, and he doesn't know you. Give him a chance to get used to you before you attempt to pick him up or hug him.

Ask the youngster to show you his room or his favorite toy — he'll feel more sure of himself if he's on familiar ground. The reason for this whole procedure is to give the child a chance to know you. Then, when you come to sit, he'll be less upset when his parents leave.

If you're sitting with an infant — a child under eighteen months, for example — you'll also need to know whether he drinks from a bottle or a cup; whether he can drink plain milk

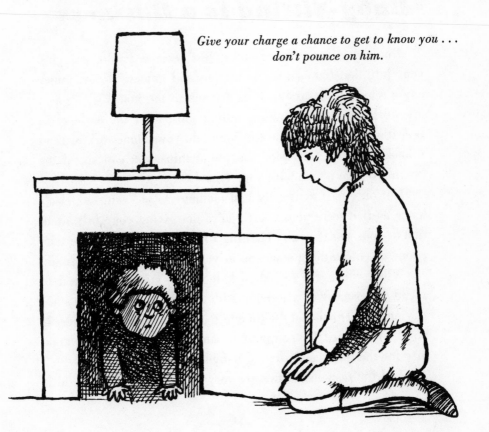

*Give your charge a chance to get to know you . . . don't pounce on him.*

or if he's still on a formula; where his clean diapers are kept and where to put the soiled ones; what, if any, solid foods he can have. While you're less likely to be sitting with an infant than with a toddler, it's always a good idea to be prepared for anything and everything.

When the day or evening of your baby-sitting job actually arrives, you'd be smart to get to the house fifteen minutes to a half hour earlier than you're expected. This will serve two purposes: Both you and the mother will have a chance to go over any last-minute instructions, and you'll have an opportunity to get reacquainted with the child while his mother is still around and he feels more secure.

# Baby-Sitting Is a Business

Don't ever make the mistake, just because you're enjoying your job, that baby-sitting is all fun and games. Never, under any circumstances, invite your friends to the house where you are working. During evening sitting jobs, after the child is in bed, it's perfectly all right for you to do your homework or read a book or watch television, but don't think you can spend the evening on the phone with your friends.

Not only is it extremely bad manners to use someone else's home as if it were yours, but you're not giving your full attention to your job if you're chatting with your friends on the telephone or entertaining someone in your employer's living room.

When you agree to baby-sit, it means you have agreed to spend the evening or afternoon with the child whose parents are paying you. This is not the time to socialize with your friends. If you feel the need for company at such times, you're too immature for the responsibilities of baby-sitting.

And the responsibilities are very real. The life of a child is in your hands, and you cannot run the risk of putting him in any danger by giving him less than your full, undivided attention.

Making a social affair out of a baby-sitting assignment also makes a very bad impression on your employer, and you're much less likely to be called again when the mother discovers you've spent the evening on the phone or had an impromptu party.

Another important thing to remember is that you can't raid the refrigerator as if you were in your own home. Usually the woman of the house will indicate that there are things you can help yourself to: a piece of cake, some cookies, milk, or soda pop. But don't take it upon yourself to make a hero sandwich — you may be devouring tomorrow's dinner for the family you're sitting for!

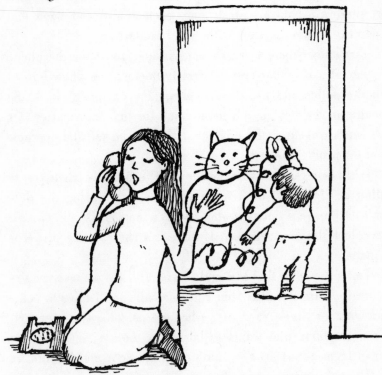

*You're not giving the job your full attention
if you're chatting on the phone with your friends.*

If you keep in mind that you're getting paid to do a specific job, and that you are responsible for a child's safety and well-being, you won't make any serious mistakes. And those manners your own mother drilled into you will come in very handy, too!

# Safety Precautions

Unfortunately, the world has a lot of people in it who are not very nice, and you'll find such people no matter where you live. Knowing some basic safety rules can help you take care of your young charge and yourself in practically any situation. Then, too, there are natural catastrophes such as fire and flood that needn't turn into disasters if the sitter is alert.

You know where to reach the parents; you have the phone number of a neighbor and the family doctor; you know how to call the police and fire departments. (If you don't, check the opening pages of your telephone book for that information. Or you can always dial the number 0 (zero) and tell the operator what the problem is.)

If someone should come to the door, especially when you're sitting at night, but even when you're sitting during the day, don't let him in no matter what he says. As soon as the parents leave, lock the door securely. If there is a chain, make sure it is in place.

Tell any visitor that Mr. and Mrs. Smith (or whoever you're sitting for) are not available, and the caller will have to come back another time. No matter what the person says — even if he's a neighbor who wants to borrow a tool; a repairman; a cousin from out of town — don't open the door and let him in.

The only exception is when Mrs. Smith has told you before

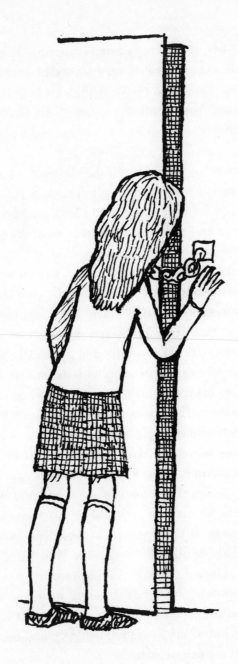

*If there's a chain on the door,
make sure it's in place.*

she left that, say, the TV repairman is coming, or her cousin, and it will be all right to let him in. Just make sure the person you allow to enter the house really is the expected guest. If it is a repairman, ask Mrs. Smith the name of the company he works for. If the man who comes to the door gives the same name, then let him in.

But in most cases no one will be expected, so a good rule to follow for safety's sake is not to admit anyone under any circumstances. It may be ungracious not to let a stranger in to use the phone because his car broke down in front of the house, but it is better to be ungracious than unsafe.

Should the phone ring, by all means answer it. Don't tell the caller you're the baby-sitter and the Smiths aren't home; just say they are not available at the moment but you'll be happy to take a message. If you do take a message, don't rely on your memory; write the message down carefully and accurately and leave it in a spot where your employer can find it as soon as she returns.

Sometimes the phone may ring but there's no one on the line when you answer. There's no reason to panic if that happens to you. It could be someone playing a silly joke or it may be a malfunction of the telephone. If it happens several times during the afternoon or evening, be sure to mention it to your employer.

Be very careful if you have to use a match to light the stove. Don't toss it in the garbage until you've made sure it's out. Better yet, run water on it for a second or two; then you'll be sure it's out. If you have to light the oven, ask Mrs. Smith to show you how to do it before she leaves. And make sure you turn off all the burners completely, as well as the oven, when you're finished.

In case of fire, don't waste time trying to put it out yourself. Get the child out of the house immediately and use a neighbor's phone to call the fire department.

If you think someone's trying to break into the house, call the police. Lock yourself and the child in a bedroom (a chair

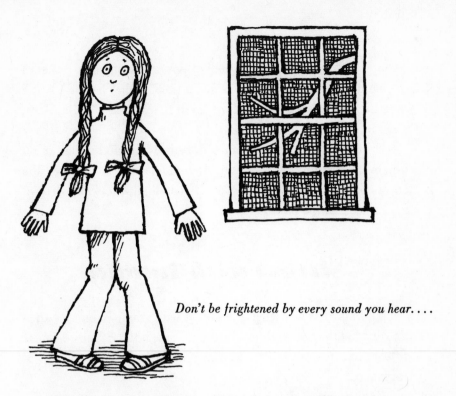

*Don't be frightened by every sound you hear....*

propped under the doorknob works pretty well if there's no key) with a telephone in it until the police arrive.

Don't be frightened by every sound you hear; each house has its own set of groans and squeaks that takes a while to become accustomed to. A branch scraping against a window can sound like someone trying to force a window open. Think calmly and you won't panic. But if you really see someone prowling around the house, or if someone insists that you let him in, don't be afraid to call the police. They'd rather you made a mistake on the side of caution anyway, and you needn't feel embarrassed about it.

Never stay in one room while a toddler — a child from about two to four — is in another room. Children that age can move very fast, and they can get into trouble as quick as a wink.

If you're in the kitchen preparing a snack, maybe you can put Junior in his high chair or give him something to play with

**21**

so he won't try to investigate the hot pot on the stove. Make sure the handles of any pots or pans are turned so that he can't reach them; it only takes a second for him to reach up and bring down a pot of hot milk on his head.

Even when you've put Junior to bed for the night, look in on him every fifteen minutes or so. At best he may have kicked the covers off; at worst he may be out of bed and practically drowning himself in the bathtub.

## *Sitting with Infants*

You may not be called upon to sit with young babies as often as with toddlers and older children, especially if you're under fifteen, but it won't hurt to be familiar with the general care of infants.

Babies under eighteen months are usually easier to sit with because they don't get around as much on their own as slightly older children do. But since they can't talk, they can't tell you why they are crying, and that can sometimes scare a sitter out of her wits. A good baby-sitting course is especially helpful in this situation, particularly if you haven't had an opportunity to be around small babies.

It may comfort you to know that a healthy, well-cared-for infant usually only cries when he's hungry, his diapers are uncomfortably wet, or when he hurts. If you've been around infants a lot, you'll be able to distinguish the meaning of each type of cry. Should your young charge start to howl, check the clock to see if it's feeding time; check his diapers to make sure they're clean (if not, change them); check to see if a diaper pin is open or if any article of clothing is too tight. Chances are that as soon as you take care of one of these problems, the baby will stop crying.

The only other time a healthy baby cries a lot is when he's teething. His gums are really sore, but you can help ease his discomfort by rubbing them very gently with your finger. Of course you'll wash your hands thoroughly before you do this.

Afternoon sitting with an infant is generally no more strenuous than taking him out for an airing in his carriage for an hour or so. The baby may sleep the whole time or he may sit up and take notice of everything that's going on. He may start to cry if you're pushing the carriage too fast or swerving from side to side too much. "Drive safely" is a good rule to follow when you're responsible for a baby in his carriage. A normal walking pace is best; you're not running a race. But you don't have to creep along like a snail, either.

# Feeding the Baby

If you're taking care of the baby in his home during the afternoon, you may have to give him his bottle and change his diapers. The bottle, and you'll know from his mother whether it's formula or plain milk that he drinks, should be lukewarm.

It can be heated in the bottle in an electric bottle warmer. Or you can put the bottle in a pan of cold water and heat it on the stove. You will be able to determine the proper temperature by shaking a few drops of the milk on the inside of your wrist. If it's hot, let it cool a little (the fastest way is hold the bottle under running cold water) before giving it to baby. If the milk feels cold, heat it a little longer. If you can barely feel the milk on your wrist, it's ready for baby.

The best way to give an infant his bottle is to sit in a comfortable chair with the baby cradled in one arm while you hold the bottle in your other hand. Make sure the baby's head is up; it should be supported by your arm and your chest.

Remove the bottle from the baby's mouth once in a while to give him a rest. He'll let you know when he's had enough by spitting out the nipple. Don't let the baby suck on the nipple after he's drunk all the milk; he'll fill up with air and be uncomfortable.

When he's finished, hold the baby upright, still supporting his head, and holding him against your chest with his chin on your shoulder, gently pat or rub his back. This "burping the baby" helps him get rid of any air he may have swallowed along with his milk.

If you have to feed the baby solid food, he's probably eating baby food that comes in small jars. His mother will tell you what to give him (if she doesn't volunteer this information, make sure you ask her before she leaves). You can warm his lunch by placing the opened jar in a pan of water and putting it over low heat until it's the right temperature; neither too hot nor too cold. You can feed him straight from the jar or spoon his food onto a plate.

No matter what's on the baby's menu, feed him with a spoon, not a fork. If he's old enough to sit in a high chair, fine. Otherwise, hold him in a sitting position on your lap, bracing him against one arm and your chest, while you feed him with your other hand.

Not only should the baby wear a bib, but it's a good idea for you to put on an apron if you're not wearing something washable. The infant hasn't been around long enough to know much about table manners.

Keep the food out of his reach or you may have a lot of cleaning up to do. And have a damp facecloth or paper towel handy so that you can wipe the baby's face as you go along.

Be patient at feeding time; an infant can pay attention to one thing for only a short period of time. He'll probably turn his head constantly to see what's going on elsewhere. He'll be wrig-

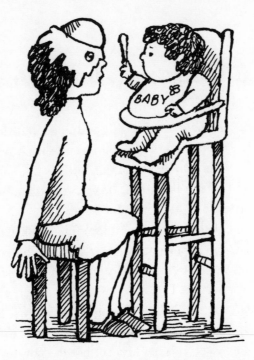

*An infant hasn't been around long enough to
know much about table manners.*

gling a lot, too; that's why it's so important for you to have a
good grip on him.

When he's finished eating, let him sit quietly in his crib or
playpen for a half hour or so. This reduces the chances of his
throwing up the lunch you worked so hard to get into him. But if
he should vomit, don't be alarmed.

Infants frequently do this and it doesn't necessarily mean
they are sick. You may have fed him too fast, or too much, or he
may have been a little too active right after eating. Just clean him
up and let him stay quiet for a while. Don't immediately try to
get more food into him — he'll let you know when he's hungry
again by yelling his head off. If his mother comes home before
this happens, be sure to tell her the baby vomited.

25

# Changing the Baby

Now you will have to change his diaper, but don't let that frighten you. Just put him on a comfortable flat surface that he can't roll off — his crib or his parents' bed is fine — and you're ready to begin. Have the fresh diaper, a washcloth moistened with warm water, and baby powder handy.

Remove the soiled diaper by unpinning or unsnapping it. If pins are used, put them out of baby's reach, but not in your mouth. You'll get a weird reputation as a baby-sitter if you swallow the diaper pins!

Using the washcloth, gently wash the baby's bottom and around his upper legs. Sprinkle him lightly with baby powder, holding the container close to him so that the powder doesn't fly all over the place and into his mouth. Now you're ready to put on the clean diaper.

Fold the clean diaper the same way in which the one you just removed was folded, and holding both the baby's ankles with one hand, gently raise him up so that you can slip the diaper under him. Pin or snap it in place, replace his rubber pants, if any, and the baby is fresh and clean again.

If you change the baby's diaper on a dressing table, be sure to fasten the straps around him and don't leave him alone for even a minute.

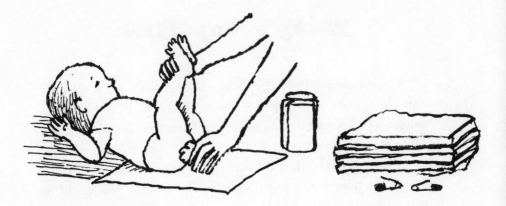

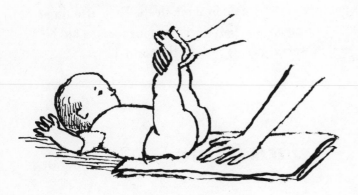

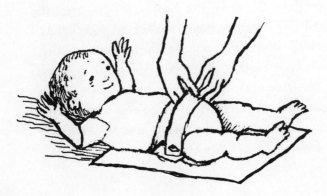

# Baby's Nap Time

If it's time for the baby to take a nap, put him in his crib, cover him, and stay with him a while, talking softly, until he falls asleep. Don't forget to look in on him from time to time to make sure everything's all right.

You've probably heard the phrase "sleeping like a baby." It means sleeping soundly and quietly. The truth of the matter is that babies are usually very noisy sleepers. They snort, grunt, gurgle, and sometimes even giggle in their sleep. They also do a lot of twisting and turning when they're about four months old or older. Don't let that worry you; it's perfectly normal.

# Fun Time

Entertaining a small baby is relatively easy. He's delighted with practically everything you hand him. Of course, he'll put it into his mouth immediately, so make sure his playthings are too big for him to swallow. Counting his toes or his fingers will please him, too, and so will hiding your face behind your hands, saying "Peek-a-boo!" when you remove them. Sounds silly, doesn't it? But ask your mother about how you used to laugh when she played the same game with you.

But if you want baby to sleep, play a quieter game. Even infants as young as three months enjoy being read to, and that's an excellent way to settle them down for a nap.

# A Night with Baby

Nighttime sitting with your babies is generally the easiest type of baby-sitting. When a baby is about three months old, he usually sleeps through the whole night, or at least from about six in the evening to six in the morning. All you have to do on such occasions is put him to bed and then check on him during the evening to make sure his covers are in place and he really is asleep. In most cases you'll find when you get to your job that the baby's mother has him all ready for bed; in fact, he may even be asleep already.

Remember that young babies don't use pillows and probably only a light blanket. He doesn't need much in the way of covers because his pajamas are warm and cover him from neck to toes and he's in a warm room. Check with his mother to find out what his usual covering is.

Don't tuck the blanket too tightly around him. Babies move a great deal while they sleep and they'll cry if tight covers restrict their normal movements. The best way to make his bed for sleeping is to tuck the covers under the mattress at the foot of the bed only. Remember that you'll be checking him regularly, and one of the things you will be concerned with is the position of the covers.

If you're sitting in the summer when windows are open, make sure the room doesn't cool off too much during the night. A room that's comfortable for you may be a little cool for an infant, so you can adjust the windows if the need arises. For example, if it starts to rain, the temperature will probably fall and you'll have to close the windows. This is better than putting another blanket on the baby.

# Sitting with Toddlers and Small Children

Most of the time you will be called upon to sit with young-sters who are between two and eight years old. They are the most fun, because you can actually do things with them and talk to them. They are also the most trouble because they have minds of their own and often don't want to do what you tell them to. This is why it's so important to meet the children before you actually sit with them; they'll know you and you'll have a chance to know them.

Some of the best baby-sitters around invest part of their earn-ings in a collection of inexpensive toys and games that they take with them on jobs. There is nothing like something new to divert a youngster's attention from something you'd rather not have him do. It's better than just ordering him around or yelling at him — for two good reasons. First, it's a much more effective method of getting the child to do what you want him to. Second, the child will resent you much less; in fact he'll even grow to like you a lot. This means his mother will be happy to call you the next time she needs a sitter.

These toys and games don't have to be elaborate or expensive. Many of them you can make yourself. The cardboard tube that paper towels come on can be converted into a musical instrument by fastening wax paper or tissue paper over one end with string or a rubber band and blowing into the open end. An empty milk carton — washed and covered with gift wrap and cut open at one end — and a couple of clothespins become a fascinating game when you invite a youngster to see how many clothespins he can toss into the container.

For a slightly older child, five or ten milk containers and a rubber ball make a fine indoor bowling game. Coloring books, construction paper, and crayons are other items you might invest

**30**

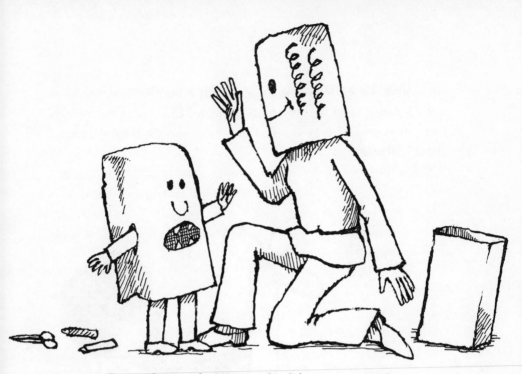

*Toys and games don't have to be elaborate or expensive . . .
some you can make yourself.*

in. Just hand a six-year-old a pad of paper, a pencil, and some crayons and ask him to draw a picture for you. If you put him at the kitchen table, he'll be having fun while you fix a snack and keep an eye on him all at the same time.

If, at the very beginning, you tell the child that these toys belong to you and he'll have to give them back when you leave, you'll avoid a problem. The child may think that everything you bring is a present for him. Let him keep any pictures he may draw and anything else that you can replace easily and cheaply if he wants them, but let him know from the start he can't have everything in your bag.

Another item for your stock of games is a bag of balloons. Slightly disorganized games of volleyball can be played indoors with inflated balloons. You might even be able to twist several long balloons together, after they've been inflated, to make an animal. Don't blow up the balloons too much; this often causes them to burst. The noise sometimes frightens children, even older

**31**

ones. Should a balloon pop, either admit it startled you, too, or remark about what a grand noise it made. Either of these reactions on your part may comfort the child who's a little nervous about balloons.

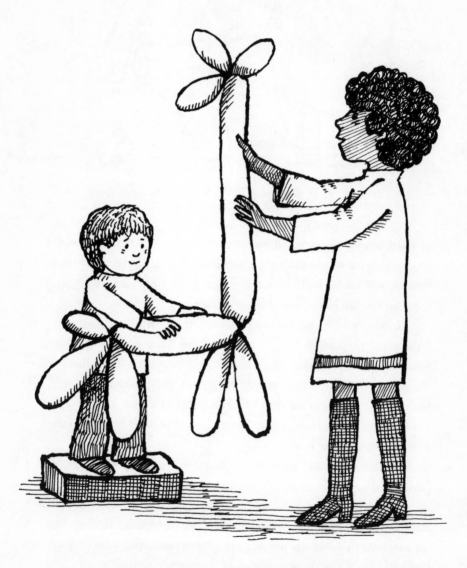

*Balloons are a good thing to bring along to the job.*

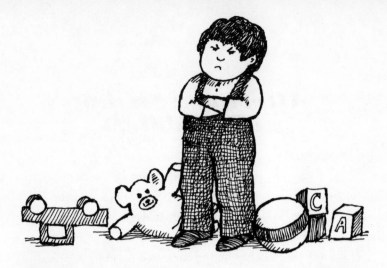

# *Get the Kids on Your Side*

But baby-sitting with older children can have its problems, too. You're the boss, and the youngsters have to realize this if you don't want to become a nervous wreck by the end of your first sitting session. It may come as a surprise to you to learn that the best way to let the child know who's boss is *not* by issuing orders, but by *asking* the youngster to help you. Children feel important when they think they're doing something as grown up as drying dishes or making a bed.

For example, if Junior's toys are strewn all over the living room at bedtime, don't just stand there and say, "Pick up those toys this instant!" The only answer you'll probably get is a firm, "I won't!" It would be better to say, "Will you help me pick up these toys and show me where they belong?"

Junior will be delighted to help you, and he'll feel important because he knows something you don't (even if you really do know where the toys belong). Besides, no one at any time really appreciates being ordered around, but helping someone is an entirely different matter.

If you're sitting with two or more children, make the oldest one your chief assistant. Ask his help in handling the smaller ones and you've made a friend. Just make sure he doesn't overdo the authority you've given him; he may start ordering the others around!

# Afternoon Sitting with Toddlers

Should you be sitting with youngsters in the afternoon, you will have to be on your toes all the time. This is not the time for you to do your homework or watch television — you must give the children your full attention every minute.

If the weather keeps you indoors, make use of your supply of games. Should the child prefer to watch television, let him choose the programs. Remember, you're here to work and not simply to enjoy yourself. Besides, you can't expect a four-year-old to sit quietly by while you watch an old romantic movie on TV. When the child becomes restless and bored with one activity, be ready with another. Try to keep him (or them) busy all the time and you will be less likely to have any trouble.

But don't indicate what games the youngsters must play; just offer suggestions. And it's also a good idea to ask the child what he'd like to do next. If it's at all possible, go along with his suggestion.

One word of caution: If it's raining hard outside, and one child says his mother lets him put on a bathing suit and play in the yard in such weather, tell him nothing doing! Young children will often tell a sitter that they are allowed to do certain things when the truth of the matter is that Mother has already told them no.

You have to use your common sense in such situations. If you have any doubts at all, it's better to say no and tell the child you'll check with his mother when she comes home. Maybe he can play in the rain (or whatever he wants to do) next time. In a few instances, you'll be surprised to learn the child was telling the truth. But no mother with any sense will blame you for being careful in such situations.

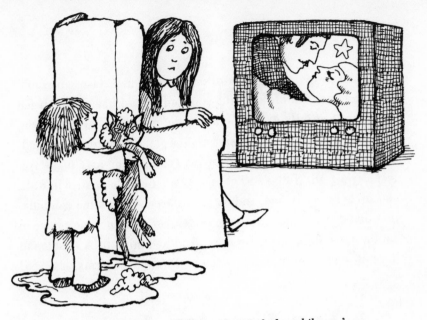

*You can't expect a toddler to sit quietly by while you're
watching an old romantic movie on TV.*

# Feeding Time

Often, during afternoon sitting sessions, you'll have to prepare a snack for the child and for yourself. Be sure to observe
the safety rules in the kitchen, and remember to clean up any
mess you or the child make, as well as washing, drying, and putting away the dishes.

After you've fixed the meal, Junior may decide he doesn't
want to eat it. Don't let that worry you. No child actually starved
to death by his own wish; when Junior is hungry, he'll eat. The
more you fuss at him, the more stubborn he'll become about not
eating. But if you simply say, "All right, you can eat it later,"
he'll either decide he's really ready for it or wait until later.

You might also tell him that he can't have any candy or
cookies until he's eaten his regular lunch, if that's the meal
you've had to fix for him. But, again, don't make a big thing out
of it.

**35**

By the way, youngsters often have strange tastes in food. Let's say Mrs. Smith has told you Junior can have a sandwich and a glass of milk or fruit juice in the middle of the afternoon, but Junior's idea of a sandwich is chocolate syrup on rye bread. Even though the mere idea of such a combination may make you feel slightly ill, if that's what he wants let him have it. After all, chocolate syrup is fine, and so is rye bread. If it's the combination that doesn't appeal to you, remember that you don't have to eat the same thing the child does. And just think back to some of the stuff you enjoyed eating when you were around six or seven!

## Nap Time for Junior

If Junior is still young enough to have an afternoon nap, read to him or play a quiet game for a half hour or so before putting him to bed. That puts him in the proper mood for sleep. Even if he doesn't actually sleep, lying quietly while you're reading to him will give him all the rest he needs. Just pick a book that isn't overly exciting. Better yet, let him choose the story. He'll be much more willing to listen if he has had some choice in the matter.

## Playtime

Weather and Mrs. Smith permitting, you may take Junior to a playground. If you know this in advance, wear playclothes and comfortable shoes, such as sneakers. Then you can have as much fun as Junior!

Be sure to keep your eye on Junior at all times. When you see him doing something dangerous, such as standing on the swings, you can make him stop without yelling and arguing if you suggest an alternate game. Offer to race him to the water fountain, for instance, or play a game of catch with him.

## Safety Time

Despite all your efforts, Junior may still fall and get cut. Don't make too much of it or the child will cry as if he were seriously injured. Remember that minor cuts and skinned knees are all part of childhood, and take them in your stride. Unless Junior's mother is an extremely nervous type, she won't get excited or blame you, either.

However, if you suspect the child is really hurt, take him home immediately and phone for help. You can tell how bad the injury is by Junior's reactions. If he cries for a few minutes and then returns to his game, you know he's not really hurt. But if he sits by you quietly or if he holds the injured part in a peculiar way, you can't just laugh it off. While children are tough little creatures, they are also vulnerable, so keep your eyes open.

Before Mrs. Smith left, you found out exactly what you were supposed to do. Make sure you do it! Feed him if you were told to, take him out if Mrs. Smith said it was all right, put him to bed if that's on the afternoon's agenda.

If you take him out, incidentally, make sure you get him back to his house on time. Nothing upsets a mother more than to come home to an empty house when she's expecting to find her child there.

You may have to be quite firm with Junior, who's probably having so much fun he doesn't want to leave the park, but tell him his mother is expecting him. Add that he really doesn't want to make her unhappy by being late — it may be all the extra inducement he needs to get away from the sliding pond.

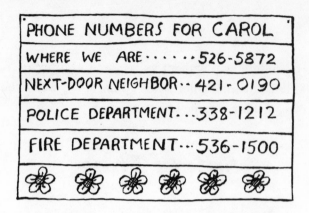

*Make sure you have the necessary information
by the telephone in case of emergency.*

# Sitting at Night with Toddlers

Probably most of your jobs with two- to eight-year-olds will be nighttime sitting. You won't have to worry about taking Junior out, but you may have to give him a bedtime snack. Here again, check with his mother to be sure you don't give him anything he's allergic to or, in general, that his mother doesn't want him to have.

You will of course have the necessary information in case of an emergency: where the parents can be reached, the phone number of a neighbor and the family doctor, the numbers of the police and fire departments. Keep these numbers by the telephone so you won't have to waste time searching for them in case of trouble. Hopefully, you won't need them at all, but it will be comforting to know you're prepared for any emergency.

Having made friends with Junior beforehand, or at the very least having met him, he won't be too upset when his parents leave. But sometimes little children, especially those under five, will cry when they see Mommy and Daddy walk out the door.

It will take patience and understanding on your part to help Junior accept the fact that his parents are going out and you will

**38**

be in charge. Since you've made it a point to arrive fifteen to thirty minutes early, you'll have time for last-minute instructions from Mrs. Smith as well as time for getting involved with Junior in some way. If he's busy looking through the bag of games you brought along when his mother kisses him good-bye, Junior may not even pay any attention to the fact that she's leaving.

## Getting Him to Bed

Now that you've gotten over your first hurdle, you're faced with the problem of getting Junior to bed on time. Younger children will probably be ready for bed; all you'll have to do is read to them for a while and put them under the covers. But youngsters over five will use every trick they know to stay up much later than they should. Your job will be easier if you do it in stages.

Start by telling Junior you'd like him to get into his pajamas now, but he doesn't have to go to bed yet.

If he's supposed to take a bath, don't leave him alone in the bathroom for a single minute. Even if the phone rings while you're scrubbing Junior's back, just let it ring. The bathroom can be a rather dangerous place, especially to a youngster in a tub of water, and you simply cannot leave him while you answer the phone or the doorbell or get a towel or anything else.

If he claims he's old enough to wash himself, let him do it. But tell him you want to see how well he can manage or that you're lonely being in another part of the house by yourself — tell him anything but don't leave him by himself.

A youngster of eight or older, boy or girl, may be embarrassed having you in the bathroom while he or she is bathing. You can compromise in that situation by standing just outside the open bathroom door. But it's often better to let a young child skip his bath rather than leave him on his own in the bathroom.

When the fateful hour of bedtime arrives, tell Junior it's time he went to bed. Go with him and offer to read to him for a little while longer or tell him a story. If you sit with him ten or fifteen minutes after he's actually in bed, he'll be more likely to stay there. If you're extremely lucky, he may even fall asleep while you're telling him that story.

But if you just put the child in bed, cover him up, and walk out, you'll probably find him tiptoeing right behind you as you leave his room. Remember, your job is to take care of him, and while this doesn't mean going along with any of Junior's wild schemes, it does mean that you have to be as kind and as patient as the rules — and common sense — will allow.

After you've put Junior to bed and remained with him until he fell asleep, don't think your job is over. Chances are ten to one that no sooner are you settled in the living room with your homework than you'll hear the patter of feet; Junior's out of bed. This is no time for playing games; you have no choice but to lead him back to bed again.

Junior has to understand that he's not going to get away with any of his tricks as long as you're on the job. Be firm, but don't

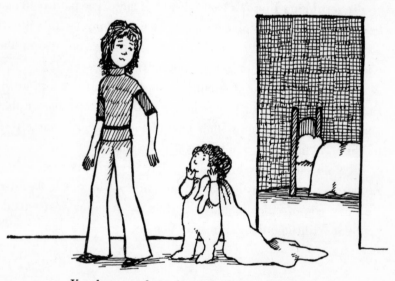

*. . . You have no choice but to lead him back to bed again.*

yell. A soft voice is often more impressive, with young and old alike, than a lot of noisy shouting. If he has a legitimate excuse for getting out of bed — he's cold, he has to go to the bathroom — take care of his problem and immediately return him to bed. The endless drinks of water is a common trick used by children to put off going to sleep; let Junior know that *one* drink of water (or none, according to his mother's rule) is all he's going to get.

At last he's really asleep and you feel that you've earned a reward, so you turn on the television set and settle comfortably in a large chair. That's fine, but don't become so involved in the program you're watching that you forget you're working. Check on Junior every fifteen minutes or so to make sure he's really asleep and properly covered.

By the way, don't make so much noise that you wake him up. Keep the volume on the TV or your transistor radio tuned low, and tiptoe into his room. If he has a night-light, you'll be able to see well enough to make sure everything's all right. Even without a night-light the room will not be pitch black; you'll rarely need to turn on a light in the child's room.

# *Clean-Up Time*

You may prefer to use this quiet time to clean up any clutter or mess you might have made earlier in the evening. This is part of a good baby-sitter's routine — she cleans up after herself and the child she's sitting for. Don't leave any dishes in the sink or on the table and pick up any toys you've brought along, as well as Junior's things. Should your arrangement with your employer include your doing the family's dinner dishes, now is the time to do them. Remember, you're charging extra for this service, so do a good job.

Some sitters automatically clean up the kitchen whether they made the mess or not. It's an extra service they throw in at no additional charge. It's a good business practice to give a little more than is expected of you; it makes people willing — even eager — to have you come back. But whether you want to do this or not is strictly up to you.

# Handling the Parents

Some baby-sitters have more trouble with parents than with the children. This is because some adults seem to feel it's all right to take advantage of young people; or it could be that some parents — especially relatively new ones — are very nervous about leaving their darling child with a stranger for an evening; or it could also be that some people are simply rather rude. In any event, it won't take long for you to learn how to handle difficult parents.

You can do a lot to forestall any problems right from the start by taking special pains with your appearance the first time you meet a prospective employer. This makes a favorable impression on Mrs. Smith or any employer at any time.

Be clean and neat, and wear clothes suitable for the occasion. This doesn't mean you have to dress like a square; it just means that you don't wear your wildest tie-dyed jeans or your tightest hot pants. On the other hand, you don't have to dress as if you were going to a tea party at Great-aunt Matilda's either.

There's nothing wrong with a girl baby-sitter's wearing pants; she should make sure they are neither too tight nor too tattered. If she usually wears her hair hanging straight down, a headband will keep it out of her face. Boys should also be sure their hair looks neat. In short, try to see yourself as Mrs. Smith sees you. While she may be something of a swinger herself, she may also

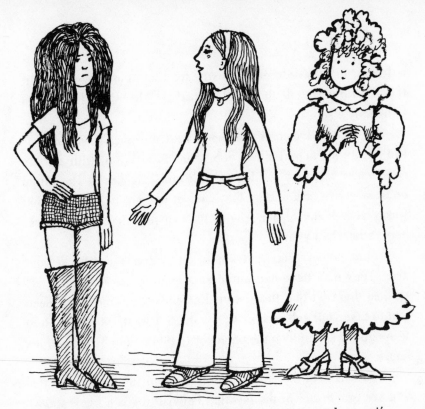

*You don't have to wear your tightest hot pants — or dress as if
you were going to Great-aunt Matilda's.
Just dress suitably for the job.*

be very conservative when it comes to choosing someone to leave
her child with.

Your initial meeting with Mrs. Smith will tell you whether or
not she's going to give you any trouble. Don't think because she
asks you lots of questions she's being nosy; she has every right to
learn as much as she can about you. After all, she'll be leaving
her most precious possession with you. Answer her questions as
fully and as politely as you can.

But if Mrs. Smith seems to want you to spend more time doing housework — cleaning, washing clothes, vacuuming, and so
forth — than taking care of Junior, tell her politely but firmly
that you applied for the job of baby-sitter, not housekeeper. If
she still insists that cleaning the house will be part of your duties,

tell her you'll have to charge extra for that kind of service. Or, if you'd rather not do that kind of work, tell her she'll have to get somebody else.

Since you have come to discuss your duties at least a day or two before the actual sitting job, you can walk out with a clean conscience. She may tell her friends and neighbors (who might be prospective customers) that you let her down; don't let that worry you. Many of her friends may suspect that the fault was hers rather than yours.

Some mothers may give you a list of don'ts as long as your arm. They may have had unpleasant experiences with other sitters, so don't let that throw you. Remember, the mother expects you to take your job seriously; she doesn't want you to snoop or to spend the evening on the phone or to invite your friends to her house.

You can stem the flow of don'ts by assuring the mother that you are well aware of the fact that baby-sitting is a big responsibility, and you don't intend to let anything interfere with your job.

Then there's the nervous parent: the one who worries frantically whenever her darling child is out of her sight. Usually there's only one child in the family, and he's rarely left with a sitter because Mommy can't bear to be away from him.

Being serene and confident yourself can induce such a Nervous Nellie to calm down, and when she sees how well you get along with her child she'll be able to relax even more.

This is the type of mother who will probably call you every half hour during the evening you're sitting with her child. Try to be as patient with her as you can, and assure her that everything's all right. The child who has such a mother, even if he's only two years old, will probably be so glad to have her out of the way for a little while that you'll have practically no trouble with him.

You generally won't have much to do with fathers; men usually leave hiring the sitter to their wives. But Mr. Smith will probably be the one to drive you home. It will help a great deal if you can give him the most direct route from his house to yours. If Mr. Smith is also picking you up, make sure you're ready on time. Being late is no way to impress an employer favorably.

If you're asked, during the interview, the names of other people you've sat for, that's a perfectly legitimate question. Answer it, or honestly say that this is your first job. But some people love to gossip, and if you're asked what sort of housekeeper Mrs. Barnes is, or whether Mrs. Jones's furniture is shabby, simply say that you didn't notice.

Gossiping about people you've sat for can sometimes get you into trouble and often lose jobs for you. The reason is obvious; if you are so free with inside information about the Jones family, Mrs. Smith will assume you'll be just as talkative about her. And the biggest gossip in town is often the one most annoyed when people spread tales about her. So cool it; be like the three wise monkeys who see no evil, hear no evil and, most important, speak no evil.

Then there are those mothers who seem to think that because they are paying you, they can treat you any way they like. You don't have to put up with rudeness more than once. If you don't like the way Mrs. Smith talks to you, the next time she calls to ask if you can baby-sit, tell her you're busy.

But don't be supersensitive either; some people are more abrupt in their manner than others are. You'll have to learn to distinguish between intentional rudeness and a person's usual manner.

The patience and tact you learn now in your dealings with the adults you're sitting for will come in handy later when you've finished school and are working full time. Learn to be polite and courteous, at least on the outside, no matter what people say to you or how they say it. Remember, you won't have to put up with it for long — you're not going to be around adults much while you're baby-sitting. And if you just plain don't like the Smiths, you don't have to sit for them again.

Some people, when they've had a rough day, cannot help but

take out their irritation on somebody else. If that somebody happens to be you, just grin and bear it. It's all part of the grand game of getting along with people. But if you take everything as a personal insult, you're only going to make yourself unhappy.

# *Group Baby-Sitting*

Some baby-sitters, after having had experience sitting with individual children during the school year, have discovered an interesting way to earn money during the summer without having to take a full-time job. They set up summer play school for children between the ages of three and five.

It takes more than one baby-sitter to run such a setup; four is a good number to have. It's important that all four have had experience in baby-sitting, and it's a good idea if at least one of the group is a boy.

Group baby-sitting means that you, and the other three sitters, take care of a small group of young children in one specific place instead of going to the individual child's home. Of course, for this idea to be practical you have to have two places, really: an outdoor spot for good days and an indoor place for rainy days.

For outdoors you can use a park or playground that's conveniently close to where you, the other sitters, and the little children live; you don't want to have to travel too far for this. The family room or garage (if it's clean and uncluttered enough) in the home of one of the sitters will do for the rainy-day spot. Just make sure you have the mother's permission to take it over for several hours a day.

What you will be doing is taking care of a group of little children for a specified number of hours every day, Monday through Friday. For this service you can charge the parents by

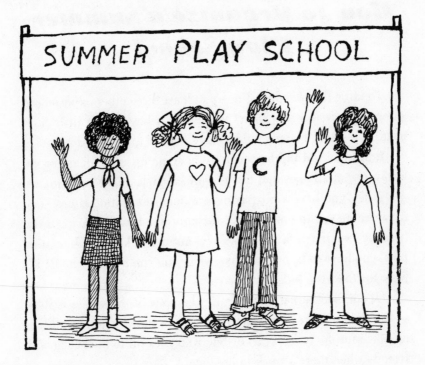

SUMMER PLAY SCHOOL

the day, by the week, or for the whole summer — at least for that part of the summer you and your partners plan to run the play school.

Before you get too far along in your plans for a group baby-sitting program, however, it would be a good idea to check with your family's insurance agent to make sure you'll be covered in case of accident. Because some communities have strict laws concerning any kind of school for young children, you should also check with your local Board of Education, Police Department, Building Department, License Bureau, and Health Department. You can write one letter, sending copies of it to each of the departments mentioned, and briefly outline what you plan to do. Follow up your letter with a phone call if you don't hear from them within a reasonable length of time.

# How to Organize a Summer Play School

The first thing to do is line up at least three other experienced sitters. The reason it's smart to include a boy is that little boys usually respond better to older boys than to girls in a day-to-day relationship. And big boys can often come up with ideas for entertaining small ones that ultra-feminine girls might not think of.

When you have your partners, compare vacation times. You may decide to run your school for only one month, during July, because two of you will be away in August. Like all baby-sitting jobs, you have to be businesslike when you run a play school; it's play for the little kids, not for you.

Of course, there may be times when one of the sitters is ill or some other good reason prevents her from showing up, but this is no place for the type of girl or boy who goes off to the beach with friends when there's work to be done.

Next, plan the number of hours a day you'll run the school. Three hours a day, from about 9:30 A.M. to 12:30 P.M., would be enough. Or you may want to run it from 9:00 to 12:00. In any case, morning hours are better for kids the age of your customers than afternoons, because so many of them still take naps after lunch.

You've got your partners, the hours and places lined up, but you're still not quite ready to hunt for customers. You'll need some equipment even if you are using a nearby playground. Balls, balloons, plastic bats, simple board games, and an assortment of small toys are all good. You'll also need a supply of paper cups, plates, and napkins, because you'll have to give the kids a refreshment break in the middle of their time with you.

Before you dash to a toy store to buy anything, check your own supply of outgrown toys and have your partners do the same.

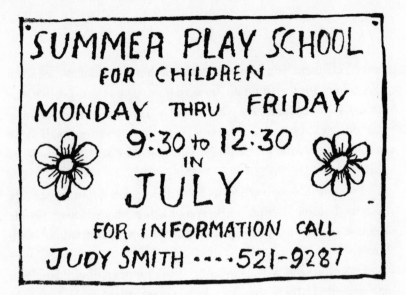

You'll probably find enough stuff to take care of your needs without having to spend very much money. Remember, the kids you're dealing with don't care whether a toy is new or used as long as it works. One thing you'd be wise to invest in, however, is a small first-aid kit to take care of the minor cuts and scrapes that are bound to happen.

The final advance plan to make is to decide how, and how much, you'll charge for this service. You can do it in any one of three ways, or in any combination. You can charge so much per day ($1.50 to $2.00 would be about right); you could charge by the week ($7.50 to $10.00 — it's a five-day week, remember); or for the whole season. Chances are you'll find more people willing to pay by the day or week than for the whole season. Usually if a child is unable to attend on a day that is already paid for, credit is given toward another day when the child *can* attend.

The money you earn from taking care of the kids is not all profit; you'll have to buy many supplies, including refreshments, that you'll need. After all expenses are paid, the rest is net profit and can be divided among you and your partners.

Now you're ready to solicit customers The logical place to start is with the families you've been sitting for during the school year. Tell them you and your friends have decided to set up a play school for the summer. Be sure to give your prospective customers the specific hours your school will be open, and the rates you charge. Assure the parents that their children will have proper supervision at all times, and that they will be as safe as possible.

You can also advertise in local newspapers, put notices on bulletin boards at supermarkets and other places where people frequently go, and you can also put notices in individual mailboxes.

However, you will have to limit the number of children you can accept. If there are four baby-sitters, eight little kids is a workable number. This two-to-one ratio is particularly good if you ever have to cross any streets; it means one sitter can hold on firmly to two little ones.

## *Play-School Activities*

You know from your baby-sitting experience that it's a good idea to keep the kids busy; they get into less mischief that way. So it's practical to make out a list of activities for each day in advance, including an alternate plan in case the weather is bad. Don't think you can keep a group of preschoolers happy with the same thing for an hour, or even for a half hour. Their attention span is very short; after about ten minutes they are sure to become restless.

Incidentally, you don't have to work with the whole group at one time; break them up into pairs to work with individual sitters. The entire "school" can sing songs or listen to a story together, but you'll find the job easier if each of the sitters works and plays with just two or three children at a time.

**50**

Since you'll have no way of knowing in advance exactly how long any activity will hold their attention, you'd be smart to plan for more games than you can possibly use. In appendix B of this book, there is a model plan to help you get some ideas. Remember, this is just a suggestion; adapt it to fit your own particular needs, talents, and the equipment that's available to you.

Because this is a play school, don't think that you have to spend all your time just playing games with the little children. You can have just as much fun teaching them the alphabet, how to count to ten, the names of flowers and trees and birds, or anything else. If one of the sitters plays the guitar or some other portable instrument, you can teach the youngsters simple songs or even start a band or small choir using homemade instruments. Parents will be particularly impressed if you can offer their children some valuable learning experiences.

And, frankly, such activities would be more fun for you and the other sitters than just playing baby games!

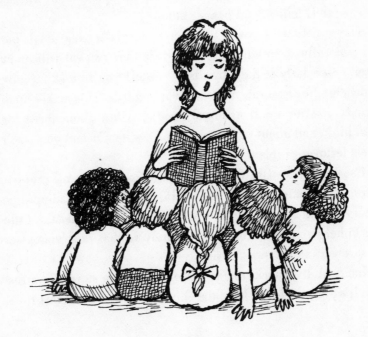

*The entire school can listen to a story together.*

# *Feeding the Group*

Since yours is only a morning session, you won't have to worry about preparing full meals for the children, but you should have some light refreshments ready to serve about halfway through the session. An assortment of cookies, either from the store or homemade, and fruit juice is probably all you'll need. Carbonated beverages sometimes aren't too good for young children, so stock up on a variety of fresh, canned, or frozen juices. Try not to have the same flavor every day; but it will save a lot of arguing if you only serve one flavor per day. Offering kids this young a choice can sometimes be more trouble than it's worth.

You can also vary the cookies with small sandwiches, but remember that most sandwich fillings — cold cuts, tuna or egg salad, and so forth — spoil very quickly in warm weather. Unless you can keep them properly refrigerated until you're ready to serve them, you'd be better off with less perishable fillings such as jams, jellies, and peanut butter.

The appetites of young children can vary a great deal, but they generally seem happiest with foods they can eat with their fingers, especially if they are also sweet. If you're making jelly sandwiches, for example, cut each one in thirds. This makes them a handy size for small hands to handle. Allow about three for each child (and about six for each of the sitters!) and you won't have a leftover problem.

Use paper cups (the five-ounce size is fine for this age group), plates, and napkins, because if you do, it will make clean-up time an easy matter. This will be especially true if you get the little ones to help you. Have trash bags handy so that each youngster can throw away his own debris.

Incidentally, snack time is a good time for a storytelling session. It's a good idea to have the children sit quietly at this time,

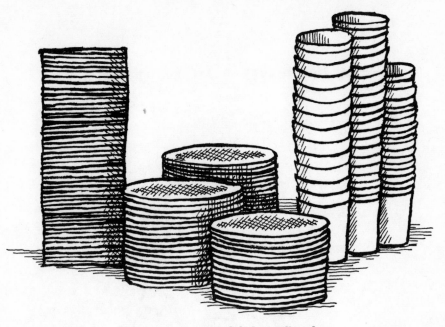

*Using paper cups and dishes will make
cleaning up an easy matter.*

and reading to them is a good way to accomplish this. Check your library for an assortment of books aimed at preschool children if you don't have any appropriate books of your own around. When the story is finished, and the cookies or sandwiches and juice have disappeared, have a songfest. This will also keep the kids sitting down for another ten minutes or so, which is a good idea after eating. Asking the children to dress up for a costume party is fun, too.

If the group is small enough, and your treasury can afford it, you might want to treat the youngsters to some special refreshments on Fridays. Ice-cream cups or bars can be purchased from the frozen-food section of most supermarkets, stored in your own freezer, and then served to the children to celebrate the end of the week. Or you may want to celebrate the birthday of one of your young customers with a cake complete with the appropriate number of candles. The more you make your play school an enjoyable experience for the children, the more likely you are to have a steady stream of paying customers.

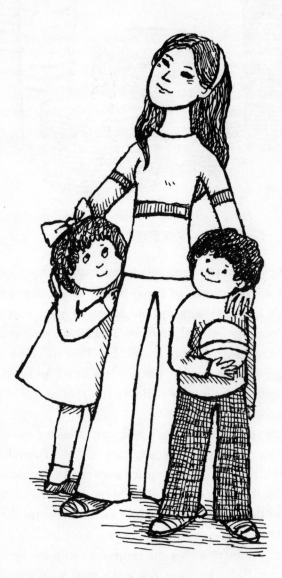

*It's rather a good feeling to know that
people have learned
they can really rely on you.*

# A Final Word

Baby-sitting is a profitable, enjoyable profession for the girl or boy who takes it seriously. Knowing what's expected of you, and living up to these expectations, will prove to your customers (and to your own parents as well) that you are a responsible young citizen. Furthermore, you may find that learning how to accept responsibility is not a drag at all; instead, it's rather a good feeling to know that people have learned that they can really rely on you.

So, welcome to the ranks of the youngest profession; you're in excellent company!

# *Appendix A*

## Checklist for Baby Sitters

Here is a quick list of do's and don'ts for easy reference. It would be a good idea to check it over before every baby-sitting assignment.

1. **Do** meet the parents and child in advance.
2. **Do** find out exactly what your duties will be.
3. **Do** check over your supply of games and toys.
4. When parents leave, **do** lock all outside doors and check all windows.
5. **Do** have those emergency phone numbers (where the parents can be reached, neighbor's, doctor's, police and fire departments') handy.
6. **Do** make sure all burners are completely turned off if you've used the stove.
7. **Do** clean up any mess you and/or the child have made in the kitchen, living room, or anyplace else in the house.
8. **Do** keep the radio or television volume down.
9. **Don't** socialize with your friends during your working hours.
10. **Do** check on the sleeping child frequently.

# *Appendix B*

## SAMPLE PLAY-SCHOOL SCHEDULE

This plan is only a sample one to give you an idea of how to organize your play school's activities. Change it to suit the interests, talents, and equipment available to you and your partners. You needn't stick to the fifteen-minute periods, either. If you find the young children are very much interested in a particular project or game, you can make the periods longer. It also isn't necessary to pair off the same children all the time.

| TIME | CISSY | ELLEN | SUE | ANDY |
|---|---|---|---|---|
| 9:30 TO 9:45 | JUMP ROPE WITH ANN+TOM | SWINGS WITH BETH † TONY | ABC LESSON WITH MARCIA + ED | BALL WITH KATHY + CHUCK |
| 9:45 TO 10:00 | SANDBOX WITH KATHY + CHUCK | JUMP ROPE WITH MARCIA + ED | SWINGS WITH ANN + TOM | MUSIC LESSON WITH BETH + TONY |
| 10:00 TO 10:15 | ABC LESSON WITH MARCIA + ED | COUNTING LESSON WITH KATHY + CHUCK | DODGE BALL WITH BETH + TONY | SWINGS WITH ANN + TOM |
| 10:15 TO 10:30 | PAINTING WITH BETH + TONY | BALL WITH TOM + ANN | SANDBOX WITH KATHY + CHUCK | COUNTING LESSON WITH MARCIA + ED |
| 10:30 TO 10:45 | THE WHOLE GROUP MAKES MUSICAL INSTRUMENTS | | | |
| 10:45 TO 11:15 | REFRESHMENTS FOR ALL | | | |
| 11:15 TO 11:30 | ALL SING TOGETHER | | | |
| 11:30 TO 11:45 | BAND PRACTICE USING INSTRUMENTS MADE BEFORE REFRESHMENTS | | | |
| 11:45 TO 12:00 | BALL WITH ANN + TOM | ABC LESSON WITH BETH + TONY | COUNTING LESSON WITH MARCIA + ED | SIMPLE SIMON EXERCISES WITH KATHY + CHUCK |
| 12:00 TO 12:15 | SWINGS WITH KATHY + CHUCK | FRENCH LESSON WITH ANN + TOM | JUMP ROPE WITH BETH + TONY | HIDE-AND-SEEK WITH MARCIA + ED |
| 12:15 TO 12:30 | ALL MAKE KITES FOR FLYING TOMORROW | | | |
| IN CASE OF RAIN | TAKE CHILDREN TO ANTIQUE TOYS EXHIBIT AT MUSEUM | | | |

# *Index*

**60**

**61**

## ABOUT THE AUTHOR

RUBIE SAUNDERS is the editor of a popular magazine for young girls. She has been involved with children's literature all her professional life and feels that working with youngsters, even indirectly, is a marvelous way to stay young. A graduate of Hunter College in New York City, where she majored in journalism, Miss Saunders has been active in various organizations, including a Cub Scout pack in Brooklyn. She now lives with her mother, nephews, and a strong-willed Siamese cat in Westchester. She started her own baby-sitting career when she was eleven and continued as a full-time sitter for her two nephews when they moved in with her.